Roseum Thornycum

I0633773

The Flowering of Aniana

Jarrad Dickson

chipmunkapublishing
the mental health publisher

Jarrad Dickson

Published by
Chipmunkapublishing
PO Box 6872
Brentwood
Essex CM13 1ZT
United Kingdom

http://www.chipmunkapublishing.com

Edited by Aleks Lech

Chipmunkapublishing gratefully acknowledge the support of Arts Council England.

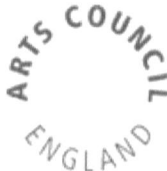

Author Biography

Jarrad Dickson was born on the 22nd of October, 1986 in Auckland, New Zealand and was awarded a scholarship to study at Dilworth school for high school and was first in Art every year and first in Art History and English in his final year and was one of the top scholars. He then attended the University of Auckland and learned Latin, and taught himself Biblical Hebrew and Ancient Greek in his spare time. He always aspired to be an artist throughout high school.

During his period of alcohol abuse in 2007, he sought getting on Prozac to help with his depression but only a few weeks later had a psychotic breakdown on the eighteenth of October 2007, where he heard voices that there was an organ spaceship under Dilworth and that they needed his heart cut out to open the spaceship and that his principle was an alien from Pluto. He spent three months in a psychiatric ward and then had a psychotic relapse the next year where he thought Lily Cole was an Arian and that she owned half of Auckland and he heard her voice long-distance talking to him from the Pier Penthouse in New York. These breakdowns caused his study to be prolonged, and he is still studying a BA in Latin and English Literature and is planning to do postgraduate study in one or both of the majors in the next year or two.

Jarrad Dickson

PLAY

CAIN AND ABEL

Jarrad Dickson

CHARACTERS

MAIN FAMILY:
EVE
ADAM
CAIN
ABEL

MEN:
GALIN
AMMON
CONAN
JIM
JACK
SETH
GEORGE
BOY
DON
MARTIN
JOSH
MARSDEN
FREWIN
BECK
PRIEST

WOMEN:
DIDO
WENDY
MIRANDA
WENDY
ASTRID
URANIA
ZERLINDA
LILTH
DANIKA
ZEENA

Jarrad Dickson

ACT 1

SCENE 1

CANE, ABEL, ADAM and EVE SITTING AT THE
FAMILY DINING TABLE WITH DINNER. SHABBY
ROOM AND HOUSE..

ABEL. Ah! - Nothing is direfully as cheered as meals
Of meet by fireside and family.
My Cane, my parents: Eve, Adam, I love.
I loving all doth thankfully do grace.
ADAM. A plentiful is present so do eat,
Imbue your tasty tongues, and pass the rice,
And broccoli with silver beet to me
In quick full motion!
(ABEL PASSES FOOD AROUND THE TABLE)
Succulent and sweet
In majesty and richer yet, divine
Entailing here is happening! O Lord!
The honeydew is softer- dressing rice;
The spice full tastes are rounder- steamed in wine
Moreover, the winery's ablaze and oaked!
CAIN. The water's giving pleasure father yet
Do quiet your voice it quivers me,
And cork the winery the cells are weak.
EVE. O hush! Do drown the ridicules my Cain,
Appreciate my cooking once only,
Your tongue does turn vinegar unsweet
And prison-fares ill cooked my food appears
To you. Is donkey-work and drudgery
The maximum you see in me? A hand's
Ability may not be alpha-plus
At chore full cookery yet loving grace
Do push my working feet and heart.
I'm horney handed Cain, I'm born to toil,

The sweat of my own brow is overworked
For you my Cain, for tenderness I feel.
Is understanding present? Pity then?
ABEL. Do listen Cain, to mother dear and think
If ignorance is a crown ill willfully, wear.
The palate's choice may change with you
I understand, and yes, deserve you do
A marching feast obeying tastes of yours,
Yet still of matter dear: your Mother Cain,
Her heart she gave us, pierced by arrows shot
By your ignorant shoves away and hate
She stands alone in tears, bewitched and weak.
EVE. I love you Cain please change to loving ways.
CAIN. A ridicule I am not giving Eve
It's only floorboards down beneath my feet
With rotting wear-and-tear before inlayed
A splintered prick inside, it pains again.
ABEL. You still do push away the matter Cain.
Ignorant glances you do give to us
And painful mockery. You've shoved
Aside your family and God himself in tears.
Adam. Religious chatter be not mentioned
My son, for our Jehova did forsake us here
To face our fearful problems down alone.
CAIN. I once was raise in adolescent age
By you my father, Jove then was prized high.
ADAM. My love is never wearing thin my sons,
'Tis only age adheres a cynical sight.
EVE. I say eat up, our chatter's at chance
To drifting heat away from dinner plates.
CAIN. The problem's not so preciously priced
While dainty animals are hungering.
ADAM. No more! An animal that waits is you
Ill Cain, an animal indeed so up,
You raise fully get leave from table son
To hither wait through bedroom walls and think
About your solitary sulks and airs.

Roseum Thornycum

EVE. We ask for little Cain, and gain yet less.
CAIN. My solitary sulks and airs? O please,
This family's as fragile and wearied
Inside as all the rotting walls around
Me here in this disgusting little hut.
ABEL. O Cain, do stop I beg; remember once
When willingly we danced among the plains?
O golden memories-
ADAM. Ah-no! The memories another day
When jocund reaps us all in happiness,
Away and up again this night now Cain
A child still you are with much to learn.
(CAIN TAKES HIS LEAVE FROM THE TABLE)
CAIN. To leave I would at any chance I get,
To leave this masquerade aside from us
Or feel my freedom's kiss arising high!
EXIT CANE
EVE. I'm fearing dearly Adam, Cain's so queer
In mind and dark, I feel the future comes.

SCENE 2

CORN FIELDS. LARGE GROUP OF MEN WORKING.
MIDDAY.

JIM. O pass the sickle there, there, hither boy,
O will ye pass it, 'tis by your tramping boots.
(BOY PASSES THE SICKLE)
BOY. O, here, I'm sorry sir I'm working fast
And far a mind like mine's affray in the clouds.
JACK. A dreamer say? This is a farmer's world,
A farmer's strain, a farmer's drudgery.
JIM. The work is tough here boy so concentrate.
MARTIN. The corn is tougher now, with winter's frosts,
In addition, men and men alike do need a flow.
JIM. A flowing ease forth gives a perfect whole.
JOSH. A flow of hands, of help and comradeship
To help us hither, thither too.
DON. O yes, agreed!
MARTIN. No more of bicker spite!
JIM. All brothers are we here: linked in grain full fields
We plough together, second praise has lost
A place with us transfixing efforts first.
MARTIN. A song we need. To sing or ballad sung
To give us pleasure, pause and passions quench
To which we cut aside the shrubbery.
GEORGE. A singing song I learnt in past, form she,
O she-
JACK. A lady? Where? Our land is starch.
JIM. Yet lands of starch and men of landscapes starch
Do need a story, spill it! Pour it out!
GEORGE. A girl was she, she coursing worlds did fall
Upon my solitude and held my hands
Up to the endless voids of loving light.
JACK. The poetry he speaks is fictions sweet,

Roseum Thornycum

A melody of foreign skin to ours.
GEORGE. O no, I speak in truthful gravity;
If having met your fairest lass agrees
Would be abound with story's gathering
Amongst these, aching fields of sunlight stained.
For up a love uproots a saddened man.
JIM. He utters truth, I think, sincere he speaks.
JACK. Yet I, my thinking caps affray with doubt,
Invent, I think, he's pulling rabbits up!
JIM. He truthful speaks, we know the feeling too,
So do get to it, smoke's ticking near.
GEORGE. The working day did drying stain the tongue
Remember I; my tongue was parching through,
And through, in thirstiness of sweat I crawled
At setting sun to our own river's edge
To find a standing fountain of delight.
So listen here, believe, loweth doubt
To join a sweeter sea, a fuller life.
(SINGING)
All boys are raised as young lill coops
Yet changing grow to be a man,
This male's now our orchard's plough
And yet, his life lays in the shams.

When home he heads at daylight's end
No dinner does lay there or wife,
A single, lonely soul, which lives
Alone in his internal strife.

He doesn't want to be this way
And wishes do arouse to find
A lighter air, a girl at hip
And children to caress thy mind.

His hopes won't be unanswered though
For god himself has intervened,
Jehovah plants a thought behind

Jarrad Dickson

His eyes to walk to River Theened.

Now leaving work at mid-day's sun
To walk towards the riverside
Through berries, thistles, shrubs and bush
Awaits a revelation's pride.

A girl bathes there from far beyond
The setting sun named Penelope,
She stands in high regarded prose
And glistening with light brings hope.

The man tiptoes on riverbank
To think just for a quickened swim,
Pulls off his shirt, his pants and thong
Then sees a naked girl does swim.

They came together joined at hem
In passionate embrace that night
Then left for lands of stranger seas
Where each man shines a mystic light.
DON. O, sir, that song was beautiful, my thanks.
JC. The musical old tune I learnt from her
And then exaggerated it in art.
JACK. Well nicely done my dear, kind sir, yet now
We move again to smokes, lunch or tea
For time is now past one, so break apart.
GEORGE. Unless thou wilt prefer an artist's lunch.
(MEN BREAK APART)

SCENE 3

LUSCIOUS LANDSCAPE. TREES. ADAM AND CANE
RESTING IN SHADE.

ABEL. Impending birds, a softer wind, a shade;
To natures call of musicality
This rest does bring my hearing homeward too,
And your new chance has brought my heart to ease.
CAIN. All warmth helps melt all ice to watered rest.
ABEL. O colours thrown by flowers, warmth of sun!
And made by Gods creative hands, our Jove!
O Cain, I wonder if you love him so?
I love him true and hopefully I praise.
CAIN. The God I used to love lays penniless
Amongst the debris of my young beliefs,
Matured now I've took my leave from him
And found a deeper, closer sphere to home
Within this dirt from which I'm raised anew.
ABEL. Again, I fear you talk in darkened airs
Of ignorance dear Cain, for God helps all.
To leaving try but he will not leave you.
CAIN. Ay, ha! You think of Jove as absolute
With powers infinite? Yet you've forgotten
The realms of negative despair and woe,
Such hellish fumes your Lord himself abstains
And waiting past our judgement day, still fears.
If God is infinite as you do claim
Then evil claims his soul as well; with good's
Own charms he's clothed yet evil claims the skin:
Hence, ridicule me not odd Lucifer.
This evil's now my babies' farce, my prayers,
And Lucifer who thrones the darkest realms
My back's abeamed with lips, which kiss his dirt.
(ABEL WALKS TO THE LEFT)
ABEL. O, help me God when beached in stormy seas

To shine your love and save a toppled sail.
(WALKS BACK TO CAIN)
O Cain, you have been led into a trick:
For see you not the majesty of God?
Does hearing miss the chirping of those doves
And fallen far has feeling missed a wine?
(WALKING AGAIN)
The devil's trickery's at work again
And you tread near eternal hells unrest.
CAIN. The only hell that speaks to me lies here.
(CAIN MAKES A CIRCLE WITH HIS FOOT AROUND HIM)
It's only here that punishing brings hell
And I'm not out of this or visiting.
So spare me please your mere remorse and lies;
In hell I am, in deep, awaiting none.
ABEL. Yet you do have the ears to hear, so hear:
The words you're mouthing now do speak no truth.
Thy god will save thee Cain and I will help.
CAIN. This moment's hell and Jove stands dead within
And painful toils breathe my days of life.
Please let this go - for homeward I now head.
(CAIN SETS OFF TO LEAVE THEN ABEL BLOCKS HIS PATH)
ABEL. Nay, repent, repent and turn to God with praise
CAIN. Nay, never shall my soul be turned from stone;
Nay, never shall my heart be loving you
Nor will the fruit you fear be left to rot.
ABEL. I fear you are demonized! This can't be you,
The serpent hath deceived you!
CAIN. To hell with you.
ABEL. The punishment is more than you can feel!
(CAIN STEPS BACK)
CAIN. Will fall again the image of your Lord?
Please move.
Abel. You shall not be a wretched man
Who lives to suffer vengeances fall to hell,

Nor lost with demons helming your own soul.
Now, praise the God.
(PASSES A PRAYER SHEET TO CAIN)
CANE. The Lord's a deadened pig,
(CAIN THROWS THE PRAYER TO THE GRASS)
Did I not give you warnings spell?
ABEL. Nay, read.
CANE. Enough of this!
ABEL. Enough of hell indeed!
(CAIN MOVES TO THE FRONT OF THE STAGE
HOLDING A DAGGER UP TO THE SKY)
CAIN. A glimmering so soft this dagger wears
Under the earthen canopy, a green
Reflection made from shrubbery and light;
This mystic moment stands so beautiful
Yet soon fully, its death shall come to us,
When shades of red this dagger soon shall robe.
ABEL. What mutterings of demons can these be?
(ABEL HOLDS HIS HANDS IN A CRUCIFIX HAND
SIGNAL AT CAIN)
CAIN. Death's murmurings of prophecy.
Abel. O, Cain.
CAIN. Ay, and deaths arrived and colour signs your
death.
(CAIN MOVES OVER AND TAKES HOLD OF ABEL)
May heaven bare your soul, for hell is here;
And this infernal hell brings punishment
With pain betiding woe.
ABEL. O stop!
(CAIN STABS ABEL IN THE HEART)
Yet love, yet love was all.

SCENE 4

CAIN. ABEL OUTSTRETCHED ON THE GROUND. IN
FRONT A SHRINE TO LUCIFER. HIDEOUS AND
MUTATED TREE FORMS. FULL MOON. STARS.

CAIN. Where art my Lucifer? O lord, my lord!
These wrinkled hands are stained with Abel's blood
For pleasure that is mine to sacrifice,
Here lies the animal for sacrifice.
My Lucifer: I call upon you throned
Infernally to grant my wishes filled.
Please answer my call:
Attolo age dum ab infernos
Tris tria num aversabilis
In enumerations in from Lucifer.
Ortus dep! Ortus dep!
I call upon your help for I'm in need:
I soon may rot in consequences drawn
If citizens who prized this animal
Return to wish the shredded blood of mine.
And call upon their Lord, whom we hate.
What shall I do? Run off in escapade?
The second's this: I am so very scared.
For everything in life's collapsing now;
Forever since I sold my soul to you
Fraternity has left - the love is gone.
Life's other half of truth has disappeared!
I won't repent for convalescence; nay,
A strengthened mind I rather want, so strong
Emotive squandering is left below
Where love and hate won't stab me heartily.
My Lord: I ask of you what lies ahead
And at your word if I may raise my neck.
(WAITS FOR LUCIFER TO ANSWER)

Roseum Thornycum

Speak, and utter words divinity hath not incurred.
(WAITS)
My ears must fail me, speak louder Lord.
(WAITS)
Will your own voice be not outspoken?
Has my own voice unravelled from your grace?
Keep quiet Cane - await in faithful trust.
(WAITS AGAIN)
O, enough of this!
(STANDS UP AND SEES LUCIFER IS NOT THERE)
What desolate of worldly mysteries can leave a child
here to rot alone? Beside a deader animal than myself, I
am left. Left to face my questions down alone, a
worthless visage too low even for the darkness.
He cometh not! He cometh not! And now I'm left alone
again, alone! Alone I stand in the most rudimentary of
human suffering. Beside death, inside woe and in the
dirt. Fate
There was never a Lucifer! How could I ever have
believed his words, his ploys? Yet his attire was
strangely so convincing; black hair, white skin and
bluish eyes. I never did see the trickster do any magical
performances. For seven years my hope and soul was
laid dependent on that premise.

Yet seven years did hold a memory
Upholding parts of truth's experience
And I could carry on...

But nay, why now, without a purpose or faith, without a
God devoid of promise what need have I of life? What
need us all this life if truth is dead?
Fate is a wish that is fulfilled in death.
Truth is dead
If I have no curriculum than neither now shall they.
Indeed
If God and truth are dead then the void is alive.

I must fill this void with my old friends and family for
there is no purpose.
I shall give the truth of fate!
Them
I shall bring them a fate Hate
Life will die voidvoidvoid
This is Eden and I must be the Serpent's
I must 666 truth love
I must . Show the ones who live the life of death.
Descending O Hosae
The truth of final fate.
To kill! Death
To cull! The tree shall die and we will be fallen
Is the void darkness or light ???? ?????

BLACK

Dark? TRUTH hate
Death death

ACT 2

SCENE 1

SEARCHING PARTY WITH MEN AND WOMEN.
FOREST. LAMPS ARE USED. NIGHT.

AMMON. O Abel, Abel! Searching forth, we do
To find you, hazy in the moonlit night;
An oddity of act to disappear
Away from family, fellowship.
We here do not believe you fugitive
Nor refugee who slipped the collar too,
We think of injury's old fainting trick
Which leaves the searching party finding you.
WENDY. Yet ho, a dangerous of course doth wear
A reapers gown at night, and darkness comes
With moonlight's climb upwards, it waxes sight.
DIDO. Aright she is, and I comply, all through;
A danger's blaze could spire up: aroused
In flaming panic arms of ours seen spun
Askew in darkened night, this jungle's thick
And waiting nearest steps of ours could be
Arabia's king sandpit, tigers too,
Or deadly adders black in venom's spite.
The dark has raised and morn is still afar.
MARSDEN. An urgency we need, hastiness
Before another falls like Corvee's fools;
O Abel, Abel dear, where do you lie?
SETH. Where be his body and where be his soul?
EVE. Here say! Away with mockery, with you!
His soul awaits in safe regarded groves
For heavenly a child raised is such

Who gracefully does gain a foothold
And gives, and loves, and hopes majestically.
But anyway, he lives-
GALEN. A mother's hope.
MIRANDA. To be humane, to yield to yearning's call.
AMMON. Yet would your heedful call uphold us all
To danger's airs of this old jungle's spawns?
A ten-fold sacrifice could be fulfilled.
ADAM. Yet wait, he could be merely drunk and hid
Away with murky thoughts and dizzy mind;
So leaving us to wallow for his presence.
MARSDEN. Ah! Sparkles do I see, a glimmer there
In front of the bracken shimmering,
My wonder sprouts this lonely sky of night
And fearfully I step to find him there.
Is he asleep?
WENDY. Ay, deep in misty veils.
EVE. So rock him, gently press for waking dawned.
MARSDEN. A heavy weight is he, he seems asleep,
Yet O! Is that cursed red I see, O Jove!
He's victim of a stabbing spree, I faint.
EVE. O fear, O Abel my beloved son
I run to you and touch the breast and heart
Which I did water, housed in my own love;
And feeling that unwiring beat I cry
Unfolded tears of suffocating loss
I will not feel again. My God above
I flocking call upon again, to help
Us damnable of spirits of the fall:
Of me and Adam, and Abel to our third
Who's dead yet soon shall heaven claim his soul.
ASTRID. Jehovah's wings will rise, and claiming him
In light full love, he will revive anew.
ADAM. My own dear fruit is picked too young at spring.
CONAN. Yet that is life, we rise, decay then fall.
GEORGE. And formed we not by God's own
handiwork?

Roseum Thornycum

So perfect seen and unashamed we were
In Eden's garden, life's own centred pole,
Becoming rotten and unplugged, it fell
A play portraying woeful men and fools.
ADAM. And now ill tell you just how fake it is:
Jehovah's not a God.
EVE. How dare you lie
And utter words for tricking gentlemen.
ADAM. But it is true, I tell you now, it's time.
MARSDEN. Explain yourself then Adam.
FREWIN. Strike me blind.
ADAM. A man who's rather good at tricking us.
Jehovah's really 'Timmy' made for all
To see, real as this bark - though not as much.
EVE. I was in Eden's garden and I speak truth
Of God's existence, listen not to him!
ADAM. Its true, all poisoned you have been by he
Above a merely powerful made-man
Named Timmy, from Italy, I think.
Eve merely finds a comfort in a hope.
AMMON. Well I did never see this Lord.
ALL MEN. Me too!
ADAM. And read his physical descriptions book.
(PASSES THE BOOK TO A MAN)
SETH. (READING BOOK)
He's docked in suits, which usually are white
To parallel albino skin and eyes;
Yet blackish lurks his heady top of hair
And usually is not seen, for he limps.
CONAN. Gods merely from the land of Italy?
BECK. That man's now merely vigilant, a fiend!
ADAM. A fiend indeed, yet powerful in wrath,
For glanderous, a ploy it's been indeed.
EVE. I call upon all humans here to side
With me and do believe!
(WOMEN MURMUR THEIR ACKNOWLEDGEMENT
THEN GATHER BY EVE)

ADAM. I say a revolution has begun
And Eden's lands at Italy we'll march
To kill and cull this man who's thought as God.
And since you've seen reality, I ask:
If any men do still believe?
MARSDEN. Be gone
With God!
AMMON. A fake!
CONAN. Ersatz!
BECK. A lying man!
EVE. You all believe his lies?
MARSDEN. His words ring true.
EVE. My lying husbands got you by the ears.
ADAM. Enough of you, it's here we part my Eve.
EVE. O? Fine.
ASTRID. Please stop the arguing
For now a funeral with Adam's boon
Upheld in this own misty, star filled night
We shall now, soon now, head too painfully.
AMMON. At yonder hill, we have our funerals.
ADAM. To yonder hill, do walking their us all
Where we will grieve our son so grievingly.
ALL. Amen, to yonder hill.

SCENE 2

GRAVEYARD ON A HILL. PRIEST ON ABOVE. MEN
AND WOMEN ON OPPOSITE SIDES.

PRIEST. My gracious brethren, I foretell to you
As preachers' priest to serve this funeral;
My heart is aching; hearts of yours do break,
So baring this with me, please do through this.
Our Abel was a prince among the apes
And shimmering celestial a role:
Compassion in the fields to teach us love,
Amazement at the sight to teach us hope
And gravity to bring us all back home.
He showed us all as prince of peacefulness.

Away his body flares to ash and soot,
Yet, soul is what we singing raise up high
Anew to afterlife's unknown sight,
His soul, please sing and thank the gift of life.
The words are at your feet.
DIDO. How can we sing
Together in praise if they forsake?
PRIEST. Since yesterday, we have been split two-fold
Yet still, please gather here and sing this song;
Not for the God you do or don't believe
But rather passionately sung to he
Named Abel.
MARSDEN. Yes, we all shall sing to him.
SETH. Yet, painfully we will not sing to God
Nor give respect to priestly noblemen.
PRIEST. In memory of Abel though?
ALL MEN. Agreed!
WENDY. It's true, the non-believers can be helped.
CONAN. O? Watch your tongue you fake believer!

PRIEST. Stop!
Believe or not we'll sing his memories,
The words are at your feet.
ASTRID. Yet wait, how can
We sing without an orchestra around?
AMMON. An orchestra?
MIRANDA. Yes, an orchestra.
ZERLINDA. Those musical old instruments do help
Our vocals reach the highest notes in church.
GALEN. I have my violin.
DIDO. And I, my flute.
MIRANDA. My keyboard I do carry with me too.
PRIEST. A musical odd group has now appeared
My friends, so sing: the words are at your feet.
(MUSIC COMES ON)
In memory.
ALL. When death has laid us down
Beside the pastures and paths,
And walks you in the valleys of
The shadow's fear, we're still men.

Shall men be dead
Sum of his friendships all will stay.

Our heads anoint with oil
Upraised in life's love, and may
You far, far away leave us
Your memories eternal.

Shall men be dead
Sum of his friendships all will stay.

Beside the quiet waters
We raise your soul, hope and love.
You've left, moving down further
And now beyond, beyond us.

Roseum Thornycum

Shall men be dead
Sum of his friendships all will stay.

Your dwelling house forever
Shall be with God, where is love
And light, peace-
AMMON. I thought we said no God be sung for?
BECK. Ay,
We did, yet still they wilfully ignore.
SETH. So God's believers now do lie.
ADAM. It's true,
And my son's funeral will have no lies.
GALEN. O, stop!
CONAN. Do stop the music now!
(MUSIC STOPS)
EVE. How dare
You interrupt the praise of Abel.
AMMON. Nay,
We promised here to sing out not for God
But rather passionately for Abel's soul
Of whom our groups do both give love.
MARSDEN. And
Now you've seemingly played us with your God.
PRIEST. O, sirs- this glitch is my mistake for thought
I here this song did mention none of God
And that-
SETH. I've had enough of priestly lies!
PRIEST. But I do speak the truth!
CONAN. Be gone from here
It's Abel we are praising here today!
SETH. And not you're Lord.
PRIEST. It wasn't purposeful!
CONAN. You know it was
And our annoyance is now overflowed,
So leave!
GALEN. Be gone!
AMMON. Away with them!

EVE. I shall
Not leave my son at his own funeral.
I am his parent Adam as you are.
BECK. Nay, enough!
EVE. I shall not leave my son!
ALL WOMEN. Nor we!
PRIEST. This argument shall carry on until
This argument is finished then.
ADAM. The priest!
He still thinks in authoritative light!
DIDO. Enough of blasphemy!
(THE CURTAINS SLOWLY CLOSE AND THE NOISE
LEVEL DECREASES)
LILITH. And who forsake!
(WOMEN START CHANTING)
ADAM. I never shall bow down.
ALL MEN. Nor we!
PRIEST. This argument is long and tedious.
SETH. Be gone!
MIRANDA. Never!

SCENE 3

CAVE. DARK. MAP OUTSTRETCHED. MEN
GATHERED IN LARGE GROUP. ADAM AND TWO
OTHERS BESIDE MAP.

ADAM. The wretchedness does seem unbearable
Without a home, a wife, or family;
Yet still, a purpose stands steadfast today.
The women may have separated us
From our own town, and their embrace, yet still
We shall return to home once this is done.
This cave is dark, yet soon shall we be seen.
Lieutenant Frosh, what are the battle plans?
LIEUTENANT FROSH. We here are situated in a land
Named Astrakhan, beside the Caspian Sea.
Our prime concern is reaching Palermo
Amongst the lands of Italy, there shall
We kill the man who thinks himself a God.
Its summer and he's flocked to Palermo.
ADAM. And Navigator Karl, what tracks have we?
NAVIGATOR KARL. The root we'll take is long and
dangerous.
Our carriages will wind us first away
From valleys of the Caspian's deep sea
And then around the Pontine mountain tracks
Which stand up paralleled to the Black sea.
CONAN. Is not the black sea home to hounds of death?
NAVIGATOR KARL. And then to Istanbul past Ankara
Shall we dock boat, and sailing far past Greece
The harsh Mediterranean sea shall push
Us safely on to this odd destiny.
LIEUTENANT FROSH. In Reggio at Italy we'll leave
Our sailing ship and move in for the kill.
NAVIGATOR KARL. From outer lands, we'll move to

enter bays
Around the area of Palermo.
ADAM. Amongst the poplar trees, in Palermo
Was built a palace which he owns and lives
In summertime, the walls are white and vines
Do fruit around the balconies and roof.
LIEUTENANT FROSH. I want you all to circulate around
That palace then to gravitate inwards;
Providing zero ways for his escape
Or any chance for magic to deceive.
NAVIGATOR KARL. And then we'll find this man and
punish him.
ADAM. A journey's long, behest we start today;
That man's old promises in God-like light
Believed we once, yet never now, not now.
So march with me, my multitude of men,
And once this deed is done, we will return
To join ourselves again to home, to wife.
So scatter out my friends, get on the horse,
It's here we shall emerge from cave to light.
EXIT MEN
How easy does mankind believe the words
We speak, they think them true and never think.
I've recently been doubting my own words
And thought, though quickening assurance climbs.
I know from personal experience
The man who tricked me once in Eden's fields
Is not a god, but knows magician's tricks.
However yet, there still could be a God
In heaven sending us to hell from earth.
And maybe Timmy is a Lucifer
Who's tricking us again to greater depths.
All men now think of God dead and gone.
With God we have abjured good and grace
And it does seem unlikely to return.
Maybe our goal will lead us to a hell
That has not yet been painted or expressed;

Roseum Thornycum

Yet what shall come, shall come, I can't turn back.
The humans are to purposed now, and life's
Own roads are all opening to a death.
EXIT ADAM

SCENE 4

CHURCH.

DIDO. The water that the earth provides me with
(ENTER EVE AND WOMEN)
Is cool and succulent, it soothes my soul;
If I could bathe not in that waterhole
Then I would drown in our sun's stricken heat.
My lady friends and I did washing try
To clean ourselves hygienically, it worked
And now our sun shines white and perfect too.
EVE. Yet nature's water does not wash away
The stains of our unfriendliness to men.
Because of men admitting not the God
We've pushed them from this town, this life, this truth,
And now it seems to me not purposefull.
MIRANDA. Is doubting now arising to your mind?
EVE. Yes, how unloving we have been of late
To our own husbands and our sons,
In whom our love materialized and formed.
And why? Is shunning really needed here in life?
Is not forgiveness what Jehovah wants?
URANIA. The things you say confirms our choice was brash;
Yet still, we acted momentarily.
The men implacably have turned their backs
And now I think they've gone to Italy.
There's truth in doubt, yet we shall never stop
Them marching on, maybe they will return?
ASTRID. On grounds of blasphemy ill made they went,
Return they shall illusions illusions clarified
With God appeased, upturned and placed in front.
Forgiveness God does always spread around.
EVE. You're right, our doubting cannot change the tide

Which all we, as moon, did push away.
I guess in patient light we all need wait
For men to all return, with God again.
ENTER MORE WOMEN
WENDY. The waters depths were chilly yet so warm.
ZEENA. I'm glad I gained the nerve to swim in cold.
DANIKA. Is there a towelling cloth around?
MIRANDA. O, here.
(PASSES TOWEL)
DANIKA. Thank you, now we're all clean and beautiful.
DIDO. Yet what's the use of 'clean and beautiful'
When vanquished is the opposite sex?
This banishing is knave, what use have we
Of empty places where our husbands slept.
MIRANDA. My bedroom's bare, my chance of sex does
sleep,
And no cavernous hole can grant my dreams.
ASTRID. We all have nothing here to straddle but
Our horses' reigns, and that sounds bestial;
My man I need with his protruding love.
LILITH. I think I need my man as well, for love.
EVE. Love creeps upon me too, for Adam dear,
Though now I think my duty lies with church
Repair, look it's got shabbier.
ZERLINDA. It needs some sweeping there, a brush up
there
And polishing as well.
DIDO. And mopping too.
EVE. Well get to it then, today as well,
We all know where the cleaning wears are kept.
(WOMEN BREAK APART AND START CLEANING)
ENTER CAIN
CAIN. So cleaning is what we're reduced to here
On earth, disgusting this humanity;
Cleaning these scraps as if it were their soul
And polishing the floor of some ill God.
Imbued in work they do not even notice me;

Yet wait, I will give them death's destiny.
Pretend I shall to be of their own kin
And thinking that I did not know that Abel's dead.
(CAIN RUNS TOWARDS EVE)
O mother Eve! I have returned from far
Beyond the deserts of Sinai where I
Did lose my grace and become lost; O mum,
My love of you shines through! I have returned!
EVE. Dear Cain, is that you? O, I am so glad.
(THEY EMBRACE)
Jehovah's love has blessed me with my son's
Return, my own love now springs happiness
Wide in every corner; O, I'm glad!
CAIN. When I was lost, I found the truth of God.
EVE. He's finally found God's own truth!
ALL WOMEN. Hurrah!
EVE. O Cain, this news grants our hearts joyous peace,
Especially that you have found God's light.
God's smiling now, I think, with shooting stars.
ASTRID. Cain here might be a sign of man's return.
CAIN. Of man's return?
EVE. There's other news my son
That speaks a harsher tune than happiness;
And it will have to be portrayed: There was
An argument we had that split us all
As sharpened steel does split a sail's cloth
And can't repair. These men did forsake God
Over your fathers, own fastidious
Imaginings, he had them all believe
His lies and we reacted brashly.
DANIKA. Beyond from here we kicked them out of town.
MIRANDA. Now Palermo they head in Italy.
CAIN. And is there anything else I should know?
EVE. Yes, Cain, there is, please sit beside me here.
For grave, this news shall be to you.
CAIN. O my.
EVE. My son and your own brother Abel's dead.

Roseum Thornycum

CAIN. No!
EVE. Come over to pray with me, to God,
We'll pray for Abel's soul, and our release.
(WOMEN AND CAIN WALK OVER AND KNEEL
BESIDE THE ALTER)
Please start the organ so we can pray.
(ORGAN STARTS)
ALL. O Lord, do not rebuke me in
Your angered discipline or wrath.
Be merciful to me my Lord
For I am faint with agony.
Turn please, O Lord, deliver me;
Do save me with unfailing love.
No one remembers you when dead
So who but you can lift my grave?
I am worn out with grieving Lord,
All night my weeping floods my bed; EXIT CANE
My sorrowed eyes are growing weak
And failing me because of pain.
Away from me all evil ones,
The Lord has heard my weeping speak
And he has heard our cry for help.
All enemies will be ashamed
Then will turn back in sad disgrace.
(ORGAN STOPS)
O here our prayer Lord!
EVE. Wait, where is Cain?
LILITH. I think I saw him take a tearful leave
To outside through the door, just to the left.
EVE. I hopefully do think he's not too sad.
Yet I'm his mum and I do warrant so.
(EVE MOVES TOWARDS THE DOOR WITH
ATTEMPTS TO OPEN IT)
The opening has seemingly been blocked
For it won't bulge nor move, please grant a hand.
(MORE WOMAN MOVE TO HELP THOUGH IT WON'T
OPEN)

Their must be something on the other side
That's hindering its swing.
DIDO. Is this small door
The only exit present in this church?
EVE. Yes, that design was from the architect.
(GREY 'SMOKE' STARTS COMING THROUGH THE
DOOR BOTTOM)
LILITH. We'll have to Cain's odd walk to end.
EVE. Yes- wait! Smoke is coming through the entrance
there!
Whatever flames are causing smoke to be
In here, we need to grab a towel to cull
The smoke for chance of lack of oxygen.
(WOMAN ATTEMT TO BLOCK THE SMOKE BUT
FALL OVER DEAD)
My God, that is not smoke but poison's own!
We're being poisoned here, and there's no door!
(CAIN SPEAKS FROM BEHIND THE DOOR)
CAIN. I'm giving you a destiny to fate
And death; there is no purpose here in life
So I am ending it all for you
With my concoctions of a poisoned leaf.
The uselessness of living has revealed
Itself to all of you, you've been dellumned.
(ALL WOMEN NOW HAVE FALLEN DEAD)
I am descending everything to death
And soon you all will die, and then all men
Shall face the maidens of their death as well.
Soon life shall answer to its uselessness
And we shall all meet death, eternally.

ACT III

SCENE 1

HUGE WHITE PALACE AT PALERMO. CHORUS
BESIDE GATE.

CHORUS. The striving legions of the men have come
Afar to Palermo from homely lands,
They're weary now and take a needful sleep.
From far and wide the dangers did arise
In heights so menacing, their fear did churn
Yet soon they changed to warriors of scorn;
Amongst the Pontine mountains dragons came:
They standing fast as gallant knights did shake
The hellish beast's back down volcanic pits,
Now dragon teeth are worn around the neck.
From there they fell upon the Black seas hounds
And fought them until dawn, they now lie dead.
When Istanbul did grant their leave with boat
They met the sea of Aegean near Greece;
Promiscuous Nymphs tempted sailing men
With beauty unexpressed in literature
And one did stay struck-dumb and hypnotized.
The waves and gales exponentially
Arose when in the Mediterranean's
Harsh sea, one boat was left shipwrecked and dead,
Along with memories of friends on board.
When Italy began to form a form
The hull had reached the sea Ionian,
There clouds do disappear and sun does shine
Along the coasts of Italy's east side.
When touching land they walked through olive trees

And at a beach near Palermo now rest;
This palace here they all shall charge at dawn
And kill the Timmy Jove once thought as God;
Yet now rejuvenating in white sands
And eating in the fruitful meadows, for
Our pleasure always wants to last, not hell.
When striking rings the bells of judgement day
While all that's cultured good has disappeared:
We shall be dragged below, there's no escape.

SCENE 2

HUGE WHITE PALACE AT PALERMO. MEN BESIDE
GATE. DAWN.

CONAN. Awake you Sodom minx!
SETH. Behold your face!
MAN. The dawn is here and time is short with us!
ADAM. I call upon the Mr. Timmy Jove
To grant a merchant with his morning sale;
We left far off our natural track for you,
For rumours, you would by our wears for cheap.
BECK. Awaken sir!
(MAN APPEARS ON BALCONY ABOVE WITH NIGHT
GOWN)
TIMMY JOVE. What dear infrequencies
Can stir ablaze my conscious wake from sleep?
MAN. A merchant's call.
MARSDEN. Where merchants who've come far
To sell our load of earth's best gems and jewels.
TIMMY JOVE. The reasons that you speak do seem
unclear
And majesty does dim; the lying speech
May always reach believing in another fool,
And fools you are, a fool I'm not, so leave.
ADAM. But Sire Jove, we are not fickle men
And our songs ringing true, please open up.
JACK. Do cut the lock, and open passageway
To see our cloths from Egypt, shoes from Rome
And everything else you shall so desire!
TIMMY JOVE. All right, this palace shall grant entry for
The group of all you strange suspicious men;
But merely for a rehabilitation's rest and tea
And not for merchants' glossy things, or wears.

For see you will my castle's fill to brim.
ADAM. O thank you, sir, we all love spicy tea.
(TIMMY JOVE GOES INSIDE)
This man's prodigious intellect and mind's
Odd curiosity is caught below
The law of heeding to morality.
(TIMMY JOVE OPENS PALACE GATE)
TIMMY JOVE. I'm granting access to my house's abode
Where we may all drink tea, or discuss life's
Slight oddity, which sees you merchants here.
Please enter here with shoes left at the palace door.
(SUCCESSION OF TRUMPETS APPEAR AND PLAY)
DON. The palace of a wizard King.
(MEN ENTER)

SCENE 3

TIMMY JOVE'S LIVING ROOM. FANTASTICAL
OBJECTS EVERYWHERE. ADAM AND TIMMY JOVE
SITTING DRINKING TEA.

ADAM. We need to speak our gratitude to you
For letting us see your antiquities;
The books, the paintings, armour, shields all show
A palace that's the seat of all the arts.
TIMMY JOVE. Why thank you sir, you're welcome here always,
Man's intellects are highly prized by me
And yours is strangely high for merchant men.
ADAM. It's true, the working class of collars blue
Are strangely dumb, our intellects are rare,
They shun our libraries with their slow mind.
TIMMY JOVE. Their ignorance is highly terse, those men
Who work the field have shot down history
And never start up studying again.
Stupidity has been a virus here
That never seems to slow its lazy course;
This dumb disease is dangerous to all
Especially to families who farm.
ADAM. The lesser ones believe our spoken word
Once said from all who have intelligence;
Some people think we do indoctrinate
But we just speak our word, then they believe,
With that, we're martyred into bounded books.
TIMMY JOVE. This conversation with your mind I prize.
I'm feeling that we may not meet again
For rarity's a problem here in life;
Because of this, I want to show you gold,

A golden rarity of our old race.
Come, vaults do hide what's worth this world.
(TIMMY JOVE AND ADAM WALK OVER TO THE
VAULT)
ADAM. My curiosity has been unplugged
As thoughts do ponder what can be in here,
A text of alchemy? A golden sword?
Maybe a stone that grants eternal life
Or can Pandora's box be hiding more?
TIMMY JOVE. To secrecy, I'm trusting you Adam.
What's dangerous can burn the earth to dust.
ADAM. My pledge is solemn in its brevity.
(THE VAULT IS OPENED AND AN APPLE IN A JAR IS
PULLED OUT)
The fruitful harvest from the tree of life!
TIMMY JOVE. Preserved and jarred in nitrate alkali
It keeps, our earth's main turning point is fruit.
ADAM. But was the primal sin not having sex
With tastes of individuality?
When Adam entered Eve and Satan's mouths
And God then turned away in his disgrace?
TIMMY JOVE. The great intelligences turn away
From what the story says, to think themselves,
Finding a greater truth beyond the talk.
I think I shall unveil to you the truth
Of God, the apple, gardens, history
And games I play like which fool the dumb.
The masquerade of god in Eden's grass
Was played by me to trick-
ADAM. I know this game.
TIMMY JOVE. How can you-
ADAM. Stop! I want your silence now
Or otherwise, your death shall be more harsh!
TIMMY JOVE. What spawns attached to your
intelligence?
ADAM. O men! Do quickly come, the time's arrived!
Antiquities hold interest but his death is near!

Roseum Thornycum

TIMMY JOVE. My death?
ENTER MEN
ADAM. Do quiet that liar's throat
With fruit of Eden's tree behind his teeth!
His grand intelligence did keep it jarred
And now it's his for poisoning.
(MEN TAKE HOLD OF TIMMY JOVE. THE APPLE IS
STUCK BETWEEN HIS TEETH WITH CHEERS OF
SUPPORT)
SETH. You've struck the masses blindly dumb for long.
Though now we withered ones do show our teeth
And what's thought low shall be evolved to high.
AMMON. We've had enough of life's false promises!
ADAM. That fruit shall poison him with chemicals
But basic nitrate alkali takes long
To wind the veins' stairway to the heart
And head, more pain is needed here, I think.
MARSDEN. I say uphold him on that wooden cross
Upon the wall, we'll nail feet and hands
And pain upon that cross will show a toll.
GALEN. Let tolls be shown!
ADAM. Upon the cross he'll be
With cries unscreamed from apples in his mouth.
ALL MEN. Hurrah!
(MEN START PUTTING HIM ON THE CROSS)
FREWIN. In merry odd occasions songs are sung
To shine our happiness, like in the fields.
BOY. A poet I did always want to be
And still do now.
ADAM. Then make a song for this!
BOY. Within the mists of beauty
In fluid tides
The soul will journey.
Levity and light full shades
Shall grant passage
To her virtuoso form.
Harps play a blue expanse

She surrenders to,
Seaside's beckoning call.
Floating towards goals
The wind uplifts her,
Her moment's given grace.
Yet then mankind will come
To pillage and rape
With devouring mouths.
Mists spread open
Showing blood and bone
Of that feminine grace.
She decays now
Upon cross, upon sin,
And men are merry.
JIM. Your poetry is beautiful my boy.
A wonderful example of decay
And loss of beauty, though this man has none.
ADAM. Upon the cross, the nails split his hands
And feet, ending wrongful wanderings;
The rotten apple lays within his mouth
And poisons, shortening his lifespan more;
And fearful glistening of sweat upon his brow
Protrudes, the sign of harmful deeds returned.
Maybe you'll go down in your history
Today, and torture men from books and tales;
Yet daybreak clear with light does sign your dead.
ALL MEN. Hurrah!
SETH. His end of life is my new happiness!
BOY. Church always was a bore, sleeping right through
I did to find a fantasy worth note.
(TIMMY JOVE NOW IS SET FIRMLY ON THE CROSS
ON THE WALL)
MARSDEN. My life was built upon you, everything
I owned, received or had was sacrificed
To gain safe leeway in heavenly lands.
In chastity, desire was gone
And marriage fell apart, secluded then

Roseum Thornycum

I felt God near; but then I found you fake!
And now? How can life be worth living now?
Though out of my illusions here I came
Away from church and steeple killing you,
And though your death on cross brings happiness
I still am grieving! How betrayed I am!
This life holds nothing for me any more!
(THE MAN TAKES HOLD OF A VASE AND RUNS
OVER TO TIMMY JOVE. THEN HITS HIM
REPEATEDLY)
ADAM. That man is mad.
CONAN. Though I feel grievance too!
(THE MAN TAKES HOLD OF A SWORD AND RUNS
OVER JOINING THE OTHER. THEN CUTS TIMMY
JOVE REPEATEDLY)
ADAM. Another man is mad!
GEORGE. My pain does pang.
(THE MAN TAKES HOLD OF AN AXE AND RUNS
OVER JOINING THE OTHERS. THEN HITS TIMMY
JOVE REPEATEDLY)
ADAM. I hope the rest of you are not insane?
ALL MEN. Kill him! Stab him! Cut him! Torture him!
(THE REST OF THE MEN RUN OVER TORTURING
HIM IN A MOB)
ADAM. Well Jove was right about the intellect:
The dumber ones are near barbarian
Who swallow up the tide like animals
And never think, just mob and moo.
If smarter ones are born outside the mass
Then we must grow, and be on top,
Then we will speak and they will do what's said.
If that is true then I need start the game
Again, and this time God I'll be, a Jove;
The pieces are all here, ready for me:
A garden, stupid men and pulling strings;
Soon I will be their God of make-believe.

SCENE 4

NIGHT. TIMMY JOVE'S TORTURED BODY ON THE
CROSS.

ENTER SETH
I've come to confess my own gravest sins
To you, devoid of life I'll lay them here.
We feel so numb at times amongst this sea
That man cant help but hurt the graceful; life
Devours upon itself with man at shore
While what lived beautiful is left to drown.
I raped a girl, pillaging her own soul
For fruits unripe for harvesting, and ate;
Her screams still frame my memory, and life
Is frightening and nightmarish at day.
I killed her afterwards, and left her deep
In shrubbery. They think she ran away.
Your own forgiveness I do ask of you Lord;
Though they've forsaken you, I think you true,
Do heed, and give my soul its pardoning.
EXIT SETH
ENTER GALIN
O, forgive our sins upon you Lord.
The men are fearful and they lost the plot
Today, apologies and please excuse.
I need a woman Lord, a wife at home
To grant a moment bringing happiness;
Dissatisfactions reigned since I was born
From those who saw my ugly face and thought:
'How dare that beast try sleep with me tonight?';
Hurting my soul with pangs of deep remorse
The women left me bare, pushed me away,
Crating their own hermit out of me
That's only good enough for life at sea!

Roseum Thornycum

And now upon your cross, O Lord, I plead,
I ask of you to grant my coupled dreams.
I ask of you to lift a hermit's heart.
EXIT GALIN
ENTER JIM
My Lord, we're humans and we make mistakes;
I know that this mistake does highly stand
Inlayed in heavens book, beside the gate,
Yet grant your love that's unconditional.
The firelight does shine with my new goal
Unknown here: I'll bring your word back home
Helping to keep the peace, your law, your love
And hope within our hearts, to help these men.
These men who have forsaken your own truth
Uplifting their own dreams of life, a life
That's made untrue by their unwillingness
To heed your call. I know that I forsook you
And martyred you to this cross as well,
But I've apologized, and I've returned,
Now I shall serve again apostolically.
EXIT JIM

SCENE 5

LARGE ROOM WITH HEARTH IN THE PALACE. MEN
ALL ASLEEP ON FLOOR AND IN CHAIRS.
ENTER CAIN
CAIN. How graceful they do sleep, beside the warmth,
Imagining with dreams of fantasies
Just after killing, torturing that man
Who now looks like a rotten piece of fruit.
I feel a newborn liking arising up
For men, that killing was so glanderous
That I do pine in jealousy to it.

Though I have come to kill these men and boys
Today, for there's no purpose here in life
As I had made all women witness to.
Amongst this sea of excessive glut
Humanity will see its final death
By my own hand, and then I'll kill myself.
Now, I shall better start before they wake.
(DRAWS KNIFE)
This knife is my own artefact, it shines,
It's like a portal opening to hell
And when it strikes, the moon shall fall to dust.
(SLITS THE FIRST MAN'S THROAT)
That man would praise me if he knew his death
Was given, blessings on the knife's first slice.
(SLITS ANOTHER)
Another's dead, now soon they'll all be dead and gone.
(SLITS A FEW MORE)
How murders own light buoyancy can lift
My usually depressive mind to light
And happier content!
(SLITS THE REST OF THE MEN SLEEPING ON THE

Roseum Thornycum

FLOOR)
O bliss! It seems red light is everywhere!
And now the other four who sleep on chairs
Expensive in their value, they shall die!
It seems my father Adam's one of them,
Well he shall die last, for he renewed
Their souls and brought them to old Italy.
I think I'll kill those other three right now
Then have a drink, then kill my once loved Dad
Whose death is second last, just before mine.
So now a drink for celebrating death
I thinks in store, Shiraz will go down well;
And now to find the mini winery!
(CAIN LOOKS IN CUPBOARDS THEN FINDS A
BOTTLE)
Ah! Cabernet Shiraz! And red like blood!
I'm giving here the final toast from men
And humankind, the toast does rise to death!
(RAISES GLASS)
To death!
ADAM. What dreaded noise does wake a man
When he does dream of saucy Nymphs, he owns?
Cain? O, I never thought you would arrive
To my own peeling sight! How came you here?
CAIN. I spoke out far too loud, he's now awake,
And with his consciousness, he'll fell death's pain.
ADAM. All of the men are dead! What have you done?
My intellect did think of plans to rule
Them all in my own garden as a God;
Yet now they're dead!
CAIN. I've given them the truth
Of life's absurdity and killed it off.
I've even killed all women in the world.
Be thankful!
ADAM. Nay, I'll bring the death of you!
(ADAM GRABS A SWORD AND CHARGES AT CAIN)
CAIN. I'll sidestep that.

ADAM. How could you kill my plans?
CAIN. All plans gush from the knave humanity
Who has no purpose here; just like your plans!
ADAM. Then you shall take your own reality.
(ADAM STRIKES A FATAL BLOW TO CAIN'S HEART)
ADAM. How dare he ridicule my purposed hand
And grind my plans to ash, as fires burn;
The floor has fell and crumbled, all lie dead
As ministries that never had a heart.
All humans now are dead, my family
Has left and- O! families are dead! They're gone!

What have I done? I've killed the seeded tree
That was my son, with all his memories
Of our old family, now all are dead;
I am alone, no humans, Abel, Eve
Or Cain! I am alone! I can't go on.

This knife shall kill the beating heart inside
Of me; and I shall be the last one dead.
What's here for me but wretched-like despair?
(LIFTS UP THE SWORD AND STABS HIMSELF IN
THE STOMACH)
Goodbye this world, goodbye and leave us dead.

SCENE 6

LARGE ROOM WITH FIREPLACE IN THE PALACE.
DEAD BODIES EVERYWHERE. FLOATING SOULS
MOVING AROUND SLOWLY.

GOD. Humanity is dead and porous death ENTER GOD
AND ANGELS
Lays ruined at my feet again in spite
To show that perfects near impossible.
Creation merely grows old to the flies
And angels to have fallen from thy throne;
My image stands reflected in their blood.
It all has gathered now, all souls are here,
Awaiting my decision, quite still.
Some wonder if humanity will rise,
Some wonder if another make be made,
For since, this is humanity's tenth fall
Why should the cycle start again then fall?
ARIEL. Because of love my Lord, because of love.
GOD. Their whispers do I hear, their churning hope;
The cold now blows again and I do ask:
What chances have I of success if each makes prone
Prone to decadence and death? No chance I think.
Then bound my handiwork must be in cords
To stoppeth life arising more and more
From loving hands so handicapped, they are stained
Of dead mistaken creativity's.
RAPHAEL. Nevertheless, look at what you can create.
GOD. It's held these people here are beautiful,
Yet cosmopolitan does hold no truth.
No truth is there: acknowledge, stand, and admit!
Now do I leave to death- I speculate?
(GOD UNVEILS KNIFE AND HOLDS IT TO THE SKY)

The silvered blade upholds the sky's own dome
In addition, it shall piercing cull my blood-filled heart,
ARIEL. What's happening?
ANGEL 3. O, I do not know.
GOD. Forgive me, yet, God I do not have;
To death, I go a loving, hating thing,
For God I was and man I take my leave.
(STABS HIMSELF AND THE UNIVERSE EXPLODES)

BOOK 3:
Lotusblood

Jarrad Dickson

POEMS

LOVE'S VENGEANCE

The pressure of this starless sky you placed

So hard upon my weakened shoulders love,

That weariness has now brought round a cold

And merciless old grudge of saddened bought;

I will so think of why in wonder love,

That you so godly made in blissfulness

Did sleep with sneakiness behind my back.

Now backwards more I step to contemplate

And trace of your footsteps on the bedroom floors;

I know you still think in freedom girl,

Proclaiming yourself out as pure and white,

Yet think of me I please proclaim to you

Of all graces, that this is love of so

Profound my heart and hand has stabbed him shear.

BUSH WALK

Softly was dowsed the path by sun

And prints with heaviness today,

With brightness made anew stand I

Aloft in splendour high and shade.

Beneath the trees sing fantails sheer!

O sweetly risen to me, that I

May join in her love song and think:

"Could nature but not heed me high?"

You've wallowed in dear ponds far deep

And grave, such furrow now and leaves

That did reflect, and tugged towards,

Do sit and lie in sleep.

Roseum Thornycum

With blue and white combined, this sky

And meadows tall now press, softly

In nooks that head, pillowed and soft

And rich within a morn's dear kiss.

LIKE A MOTH IN SILENCE

I, flying like a moth in silence

Struck a heavenly note upon your lips,

Beholding all within those feathered pupils

Dreams stirred gales again,

A knocking of my current royal place

Into the shadowed phantom-land that fleeing cries your name.

Before you I draw my loss of breath,

And blowing a kiss upon that sighing wind

Lost is my soul,

Fleeing the moment for heaven on such lips

It fell apart and died beyond her altar.

O purity, find my heart;

Within lays heaven and all light;

Roseum Thornycum

Therefore, lose yourself and bear no torch

For petalled radiance is all which shines.

Parched, the seven seas crumbled me,

In amidst my luck-lost wheel of time

All which over the water was drowning,

Life has snuffed its source and cried,

And I myself kissed death.

Yet with a blooming eventide

You lit the stars, earth grew again.

And missing sea and dust the flowers kissed

The newborn universe,

Still emptiness, cast its whisper close

Came stark and cold before your moon.

EYES OF ANOTHER

This love is rising higher

Gliding over who I've seen,

She takes me up to this blue expanse

Amongst the emblems of joy.

I'm feeling hope again

And love is pouring from my veins,

I am the wind that is drifting

Through your love and with your heart.

REFLECTIONS ON AN ANGEL

The earth brings forms

Awakening from slumbered sleep,

To my own bird call

The mother does express.

When fallen have we all

Away from hoping, life and love,

The earth shall wake again.

Her grace did give another

Beckoned to my call

Of sorrow and suffering.

And angels here again.

I lift myself to love

And her shrine is becoming my all.

Jarrad Dickson

My words are failing to express

My heart, now mind is King

And love is hidden under

Cover of tomorrows.

She is my absolute and pain will rise, bite

Or capture me if I lose her touch.

I'll never leave her now,

Eternity will cup us.

The lands of tomorrows are unwrapped

And she has gone far away.

Her leave was taken early

Yet horror stirred my heart.

The horizon now cups her name

While I am left without her form.

The sweeter fays will come

Roseum Thornycum

For they have already kissed

And new love stirs my lips.

DRAMA CLASS

Strangely yearning for liberation

A pull home or an ego's sign.

Emotional tendencies hidden in darkness,

Drained of my evolutionary instincts.

Thinking of this again,

Unable to concentrate.

Decisions are unconditional with

The machines ticking

For their embraces,

On the other side.

Pacified now, emotionally filled,

Such cold and frozen eyes,

A pull back.

Roseum Thornycum

Praising my reflections

For softening this insanity,

Daylight sparks

This uplifted breeze from the gulley,

Not forever though darkness comes soon.

The queen's reflection exposes its layers:

Silver stripped away.

A hidden face discovered, beneath the reflection,

Exposing its narcissism.

The multitude of signs

Infinitely stretching down the gulley,

Neon for humanity finally lit up by my own eyes.

Its solitude,

Exposed and thought over,

Yet, gravity still shall hold me.

But the sun shall shine.

MY OWN HAND

Wrapped in white

The innocence of a lullaby,

Softly sung by my own ego

To soothe the truth of need.

Hiding from the flames

A baby in a cot,

Totally oblivious, wrapped in white,

As the lullaby drifts down from above.

Unwrapping these sheets

The hand loses its strength,

Finally failing its hold

Withering once again to dust and ashes.

Jarrad Dickson

I step forward

The fire now roaring white, orange and red,

Beautifully lighting the circular faces of possibilities;

While the heat devours my cloudy senses

Until only the truth of need remains.

PEBBLE

Still waters, silently calm,

Unmoving, temporarily shut down;

Familiar drops, echoes of the dead, dripping.

Circulating around me, pulling me, enveloping me, a hand for the long road ahead.

Flooded, temporarily shut down;

Beneath the circles,

Voices of the dead, influencing,

Giving thought to the droplets.

Into the clouds sombre gaze

A weather Godcirculating around,

Pulling this, enveloping this,

A mind for the long road ahead.

Petrified, a stone in the river

Amongst the banks burden,

Debris synchronising?

A companion for the pebble's road.

Lost again and disintegrating;

A powder of the earth

Forming, condensing into rock.

Lost again and disintegrating.

Alone and tired,

Cold from the river's stormy waves

And reckless sacrifices, negatively cynical.

Upon the pebbles stormy surroundings

A starless night brings new drops, unfamiliar,

Echoes of the living,

A friend for the short road.

Roseum Thornycum

3?

The soft feathers plead their welcome

Waiting for time to reach two or one.

Winter frosts cover my conscience;

Greeting the dragon from the well.

Assorted arrays,

Surrendering to my inability.

Joining the line

As history speaks the future. Maybe.

Till the ladder is dropped

By my reflections.

Choosing our duty

Jarrad Dickson

To be human: As time ticks from two to one.

Surreal drifts on the well's surface,

An opening beyond the circle.

Choosing our duty to be human;

To live in the circle;

To walk the line

Under the influence?

Drifting from opposite to opposite.

All too human or not.

Maybe.

PLAIN

Forever dormant i lie here trodden over, laid bare.

Down the wind at the bottom of that cessless pit,

No hope lies within my breast.

Forgetting crowds who live to rise, i rest

Nestled safely within this nest.

Amongst a stormy sea of conformity

That starry sky above holds nothing for me.

Left to wither, left to rust,

This was a life that never had anyone.

THE NATURE OF CHOICE

"Pain" you said will

Now be left behind, yet onwards moving

Throughout hell and heaven's sky

To pain again! Arising grievances to high

Under abandonment; in stillness, so still

I ask "Is the journey worth its living price?"

Keep stiller my precious and more stiller through it,

Revel in release until your through with it.

'Tis unlikely such bars, such chains

Are held not by me

But by those who wish to be free!

Revelling in happiness glorified

And guarded; O life's family

Roseum Thornycum

Holding back this door to darkness!

Sing it! O sing it! To the masses blindly!

Knockingly knock on death's door unkindly!

"Could this be drama's song?"

I say; gravity shedding along

My blood in a pained crusade

So fake, cutting the fountain parade

Of life to nil with plastic,

Opiate for suicidal masses?

The garden has grown, grown up so strong!

Trim it! Cut it! Cull and slice it small!

This body is pushed 'aside'

As i contemplate suicide

Alone, released so succulently

Dead on that martyred throne;

Abiding today and dead tomorrow

Morn, wallowing's end is prophetically seen.

The death parade! O the death parade

Is near! Sing does the dear child leaving earth in tears!

CYCLIC

A sun shines

Emitting its rose-like beauty...

I feel the sensation

A whirlpool stirring my depths...

To the surface i rise

Awaiting the hopeful revelation...

A grey figure sits

Above a field of placid daisies...

Pleasure is minimal

With darkness tracing me back to the cave...

The hammer is falling

And darkness reveals unlasting comfort...

FORGOTTEN CHILDREN

His hold like wind

Molding me to its cast...

Their sevenfold stare

Bowing my head to their clasp...

Her golden gesture

Living repeatedly in the sky...

That shed rope

Pulling me into that presentable light...

Positions of glory

Driving me upwards to reach the sun...

Roseum Thornycum

O! Forgotten children!

What have we become?

AWAITING

Lit is the golden light

Illuminating the sun's dawning,

Awaiting do I in eager might,

Made anew yet in eternal cycles

Mimicking the new in joy evolving to sorrow

'Sun is risen, light deteriorates the arrow,'

Awaiting revelation do I dying and narrow.

Shall it be unfolded, undone optimistically?

Or cycle could I be turned down downwardly?

O father please turn to me!

Here i am, always reaping, weeping;

An illusionist wish heavenly so yet churn o'er churn I
sow;

Time folds in and light is seen.

THE CYCLE OF OBSESSION

In the sea

Dwelling in myself,

Scared of all possibilities

Sparkles form as a feminine source marks its time:

The hook.

Hooked,

Raises upwards

A placid Venus becomes divine

Creating a goddess of a mind,

Luring with perfection, held until kissed.

Salty,

Mars opens his eyes.

Kissing myself while illusion comforts me

In the mirage falling as mind is left

Behind; left with Venus' primordial slime.

Collapsed mind

Mirage pushed aside,

A place of femininity

Nature churning as she transmutates this glory,

Venus.

THE EMERGED PARADIGM

Sleeping on Venus's steeple

In a garden, while she

Transpires to his crown.

The coils untangle:

Whispering.

Fruit is below;

Descending to the people

Awakening from their shangles,

A new desire:

Red.

Fuelled by a she-wolf

Pushed into ploughing fields

Red lifts green and shows brown,

Civilisation made anew.

Awake on Mars steeple,

Found gold in the purest.

Stuck in the Coliseum

Beasts roaring for death of a few;

He looks up

At a fake gold crown.

THOUGH ART FORGOTTEN

She stands alone and unforgotten

Flared such angelic wings which bliss had spoken;

Withered and weakened I proclaim:

"O Elias! Does she salvage me or need I cry in vain?"

Forth such golden invitation shone

Let pleasure break heavenly skies to find

A rest, with storing in grace you'll need not despair!

Glory such as never revealed to thee

Lying here such infinite sparks of eternity,

Mine yet breeds rot and despair

Falling fragments of truth giving a six foot lair,

Left behind stale becoming knave

Angelic above shining she so craved!

Though art forgotten I collapse broken and withered in pain.

D

Here

In this moment,

I exist.

Devoid of circles

And also within.

My body will fail the road

And my will will fail the ladder.

I may be glorified.

I may be petrified.

The Crone:

It never leaves,

Roseum Thornycum

Never has been or not been.

Lingering on the outskirts with these collective by-

products manifesting in my brain,

My head creeps closer to my grave.

I wake up

Though the dream stays with me.

A reflection speaks its whisper

And my eyes see through it.

Pushed back to the delusional gulley,

And pushed back to the gulley of need,

Just to survive.

A realization,

Still delusional.

Though conscious of these by-products,

Conscious of this Hawk's needs.

MUSIC BOX

Fairies hide within this wooden square

Speaking of Angels; majestic elves and feasts;

Spires of Arturian lairs!

O! High heights of musical delights!

High o'er solemn lands of despair

Below thee tortured angels! Covenant of beast!

Twisted toots never placid, never rest,

Flee child leave this Luciferian lair!

Bloody bodily antiquity growing innocence near

With rising libido seen by Shires eye;

Halt! – unorthodox affairs,

Purity! Purity! Atlantea herself climaxed in growing despair.

THE LADDER AND THE GREAT COLLAPSE

The ground slips away...

Leaving my senses, leaving.

The moment withers away...

The past now,

Fading back to the open air.

The searchers take up their sticks

Trailing through the barren lands.

Breathing reason for sufficiency.

Beauty.

The arrangement of complex,

A human form,

Complication, sophistication.

Roseum Thornycum

The ladder of infinity,

Reasoning or transcending each step to the impossible,

I fail and fall.

The deep feels unbelievably arctic.

My reason deteriorates,

Time folds in.

Breathing misty air,

A thousand sounds take form;

O the beauty.

THE GRANDPARENTS

Youthful lights of Suns retreating

Westwardly to descend within antiquity

Left such youth to fear, to jeer

Now dark convalescence sides in historic evening.

A moon of old shedding its story.

Say they did such a two revelation murmuring:

"Veils and walls risen that our turning

Witches bracken left to pasts unlearning,

A completely classic land so grand, so fair,"

Though present graced in Dog's despair,

Decadent breeds this night continuing.

Fades forgotten couple with echoing piano blue

Dripping sorrow touching blackesque.

Roseum Thornycum

If time is linear history shows a bill:

"Broken and hungry! The moon explodes in shrill!"

The nobility of we now lie in wretched debauchery

Leaving a land graced to the next continuing.

Jarrad Dickson

INNOCENCE

The tufts so laid out white and free

With touch of soft women's beauty,

Uphold to me in grandeur tall

And soft, flowers amongst the world.

Such light so pure and bright arisen,

To now witness loves shining wings

Of heaven's golden canopy.

Shall innocence be vouchsafed near?

That freedom with such innocence

And golden lightness arising up!

The morning sun grants love so pure,

Which I am but one captor to

Its wings of whiteness innocence,

The pure will shine of love made free.

THE NIGHT'S DEW

Such softness raised to me in restfulness

Down low i tread, this nights gateway upon

You, me, arising up, up, the light of sleep!

Fountains of lights splendour i move onwards.

And so fragile, the brittle wearing cold

Of life, to move and shy like i was free?

These goals to sow, dreaded meaning or pain

That wear me low, let reaped unsow.

Arising forms that spoke so dear now wear

The dew of night, sweet gravity and stars

Lift on my robe with feathers now in bed;

In starry seasons loud in fright, i sleep!

Jarrad Dickson

The youth of her in marvelled might stand I

In coupled dreams, the ship now docked rainbowed

With magic touch so free, now I can be

The one the stars do wish on down freely.

METAMORPHOSIS

Though sweat such worms did display

Abounding grievances so commercial flavescent and fake;

Confidant webs in spiders' decay.

Deviant mall housed this worm so hellish

Lied and raised with thee slugs of selfishness!

Cocooned so Sodom with such dirty ash

Lifted worm now phoenix to heaven's Reich of calm.

Humane marks fade from whippings of lash

Stings so Sodom laid bare beneath balm.

Winged butterfly singing songs so sweet

All the while shedding skin and rising up complete!

Dive be deepened from the stale and decadent thrill,

Disappointing creature release your mighty will!

Jarrad Dickson

THE DEATH OF A GOD

The price I paid was high

To find it, striving for God

To truth and did I find it?

Was not my life spent in utter distress

Driving for esoteric mightiness?

Touch I did on the universal

Centred heart of life:

Beings saw I of myths divine

Intransigent with changing time;

Though when I put my finger in

Did it not all turn to strife?

Now has life no centred

Godly heart to give?

My past now martyred

On a blurry cross so relative that need I continue?

Roseum Thornycum

The future is standing theatrical in splendour,

Yet little workmen deconstruct stagecraft

With mirth so hideously draft

That need I continue?

A MYSTIC'S DREAM

When all begin to feel the breath

And beauty of the stars;

That expanse of moonlit depth

Offering no bonds nor answers;

Now it begins to be, to feel

Night vanishing the becoming

And to those to whom we shall kneel,

Revealing a union with the heart of all

Existing, granting our souls a liberating fall

Where wholeness is felt and the absolute is all.

-Infinity with love and heart-

Eternal in darkness and mind- opposites are one;

Healed the struggle is; all is one 'Tis done!

Such union with freedom: O passageway to love
eternal.

DELUSIONAL

Waiting,

Repetitive squares sitting.

Still yearning for the left,

Desperate for a reflection of difference.

Maybe each star holds its story

Yet normality is an itch,

Worshipping the Genie from the bottle.

Reflections are synchronised,

A starry night of illusions.

Daylight comes,

Though nightfall still claims its hold.

How pitiful.

Roseum Thornycum

STAINS

Shallow and weird we all fall from our blessing skies,

Through its own storm of hell we arose to be missed

Down to another in loving and mystical of lands.

Shepherds of fate are becoming too harsh and we'll slip.

Daisies will scent and uplift and I'll think I'm free.

Weathered and rotting the bottom is dying in deaths

Blooms as a flower I plucked up before it had lived.

Deepening stars of its life in my past do not leave.

Scraping is what is awake and her lullaby pains

Fear into bone as a flight is upgone and upraised.

Scent of its life are around as torment in my grave.

Taken again to a lighter of day we are blessed

Gracefully as youths who do teach all our hearts to be loved

Though all descend it again and we shall be in hell.

A CHANGE OF PLACE

The geometric lines that structured me

Are leaving for the sea,

When tides do turn

What was built is lost in becoming.

Arising waves now crash our shores

Uncharted or explored

And soon the ship shall reach the port.

Throwing a sinker in too deep

Shall grant a new, new mystery,

One which may damage my heart.

The ocean sparkles again

And life shall grow within.

THE RULES OF YOUR VACATION (SUNG BY COFFINS)

And once being alone in misty days

Of emptiness, abandonment, and fate

We were; the cold those rivers spoke was harsh

And succulently dark, it ploughed my depths.

However fires now roar like lions now

Imbuing me inwards, a social nest;

The spiders web of sociality

Attaining gracefully my dear soul.

Perfect bared their golden faces here:

Amongst illuminating light she's seen

Original in my imagining,

Like all the rest she is so beautiful.

Roseum Thornycum

The sun's crept closer, tall in height, a star

Which beckons all who've worshipped upon its flesh

Hence fuelling its own energy, a fake,

Now wands have been upraised.

We've all been leaving pain behind us here

To touch the sky's angels once we've tried;

We're happy here, away from life's true eyes.

And will alone stand up? Today?

The dimming fins lost it flame, its heart;

Away the creatures move backwards to act

And softly sing away the tune, to dust;

Yet hearts were beating and she is alive.

MOVING FORWARD

Moving forward

To see myself in the mirror,

I'm hoping, praying

For picture perfect

And yet I see clouds

And stormy weather.

I'm amongst the humans

And they are beautiful

Yet I am not.

My self-esteem is looped

Into circles as I look again

To be free or caged.

I am human and I am scared.

HAPPINESS

The mountain eagle awaits

Me to see the dawning sun,

I feel my eagerness at once

To live and breathe a human.

His eyes do shine

And he does smile in happiness

To me in hope at once.

My happiness is shining like an eagle:

Freely it climbs

The tunes of passion

While breathing absolute love.

PAIN

The loss has lost its loss

And gain has gained its gain.

An urgency's need brings me here

For myself.

Not for you.

I am awakening from pain

For myself.

Not for you.

I have carried on in this life

For myself.

Not for you.

This life of mine will meet death

For you and

Not for myself.

Roseum Thornycum

Yet now contemplating

In my woeful boat

I realise I am scared.

When everything begins

To disappear

I shall appear

And I shall hurt.

The sky has bled for me

To make me stay.

Yet now I see it merely rained

Because of the water's dew.

I shall carry on with garden work

Lost in the sleepy tides of fearful cradles.

The loss has lost its loss

And the gain has gained its gain.